To Peter, Anna, Tiff, Michael, Sara, and David.

Thank you for your supportive prayers when Mom was sick!

Enjoy!

Mother

What Happened When Mommy Got Cancer

Written by **Mathuin Smith**
Illustrated by **Ranya Ghazaly**

Published by
Waguni LLC
3688 Yorktown Village Pass
Annandale, VA 22003

Special thanks to BAN for their support.

ISBN 978-0-9853851-0-1

FIRST EDITION 2012

A portion of the proceeds from the sale of this book will go
to the Conquer Cancer Foundation of ASCO (American
Association of Clinical Oncology).

PREFACE
By Jocelyne Smith

It is such dreadful news for anyone to learn that they have cancer. It is even more so when a mom with young kids is diagnosed with this disease. This is my case. All I could think of when I was diagnosed with Inflammatory Breast Cancer were my small children; my six-year-old son Mathuin and my three-year-old daughter Sasha.

My first and immediate resolution was that I would do my absolute best to ensure this battle with cancer would somehow impact their lives positively or at least keep them the joyful, innocent and happy kids they deserve to be.

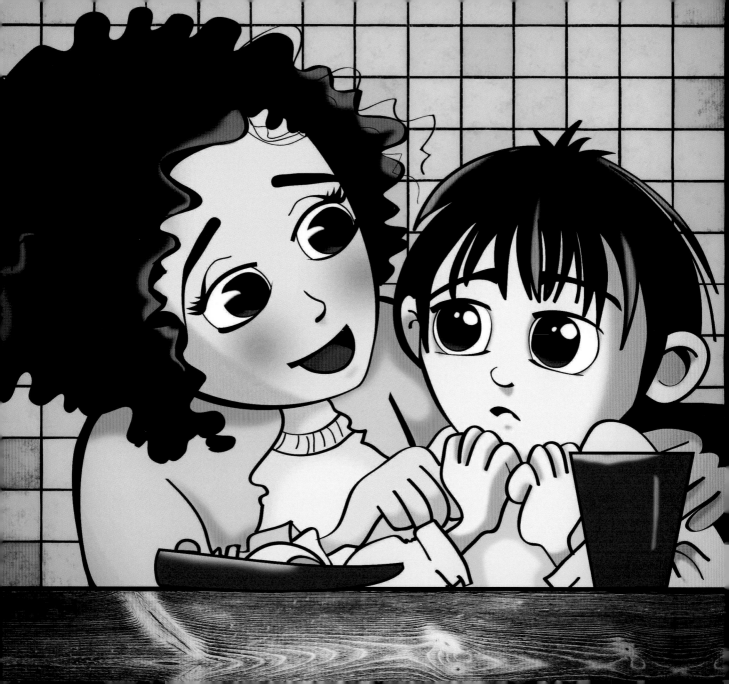

Hi! I'm Mathuin (MATH-win). I want to tell you about my mommy when she got sick.

When my mom told me she had cancer, I didn't know what that meant so I felt a little bit scared and I started crying. I asked her "What does that mean?"

So, my mommy told me that having cancer means that she will be sick for a while. Some days she will feel good and will be able to take us out and play with us. We can go to the backyard and play ball and do everything we usually do.

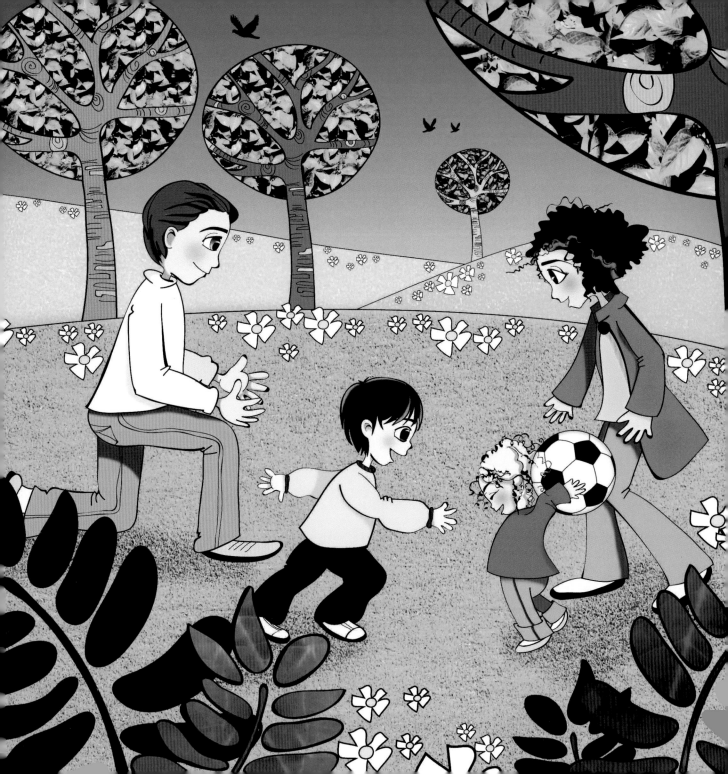

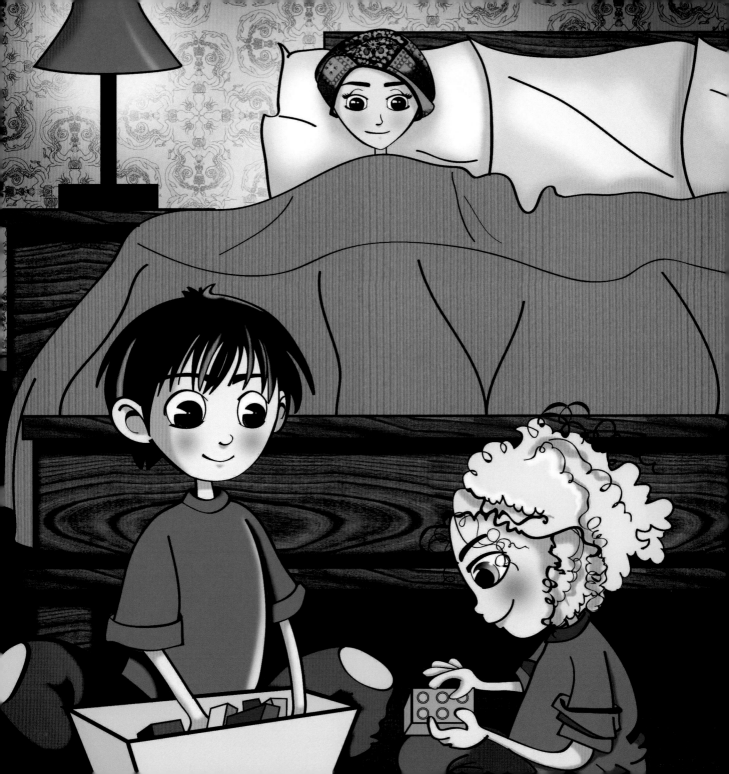

But sometimes she will be too tired and we will have to come to her bedroom and play quiet games. Mommy also told me that her hair was going to fall out.

We did not want to see her hair fall out. So, we decided to have a HAIR CUTTING PARTY. My uncle, the best hair cutter ever, came to our house. He cut my mom's hair first, my hair second, and my little sister Sasha's hair last. It was fun!

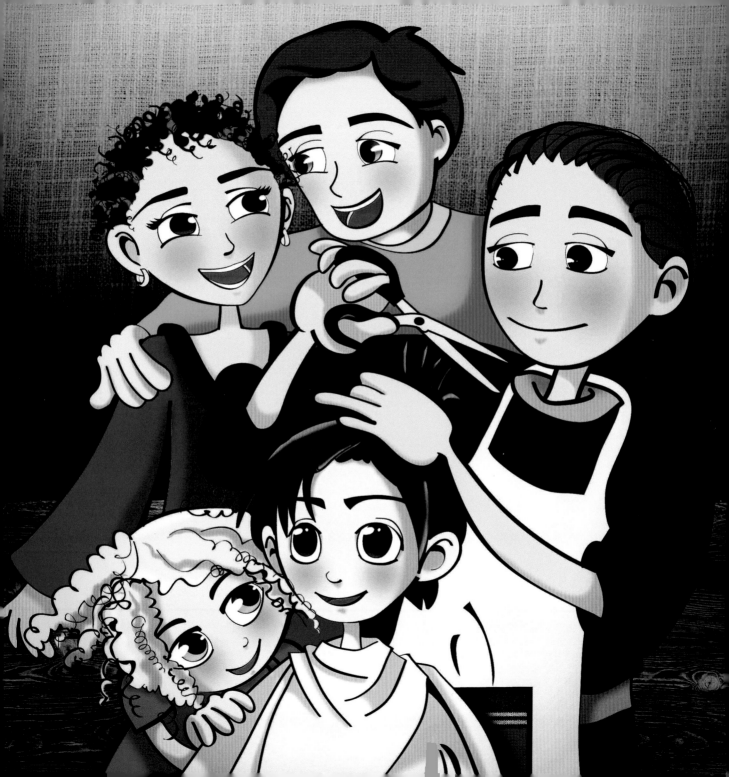

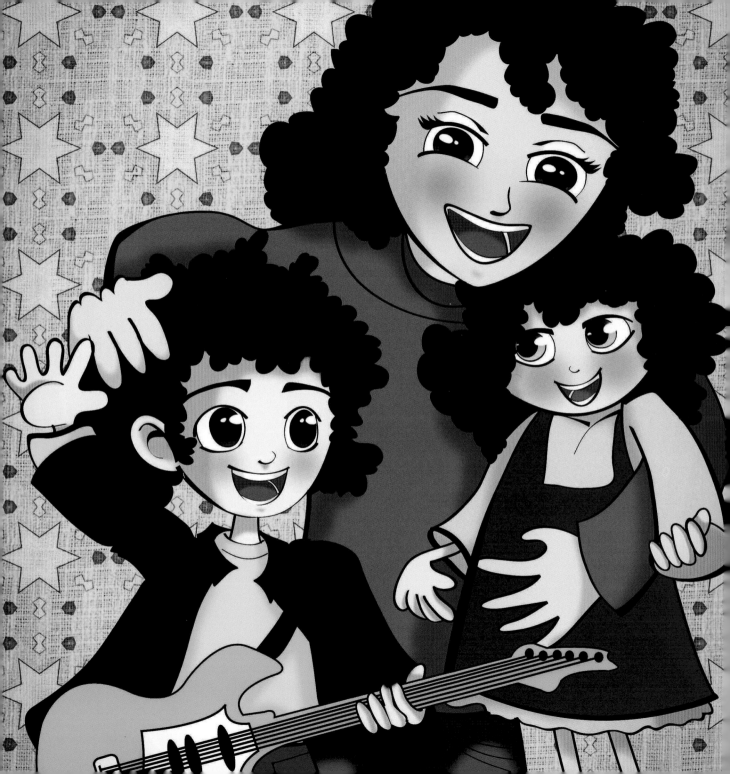

On another day, Mommy came home with a surprise...new hair on her head! It was a wig and it made her look so different! She had bought several of them. I put one on my head and Sasha tried the other one. We thought we were rock stars.... YEAH!!!

Now Mommy's hair is gone and has not grown back yet. I love to rub her head and I think it makes her feel good. I have always loved it when she gave me a back rub before I go to sleep. Now, it's my turn to give her rubs. I like to do that when she is not feeling well.

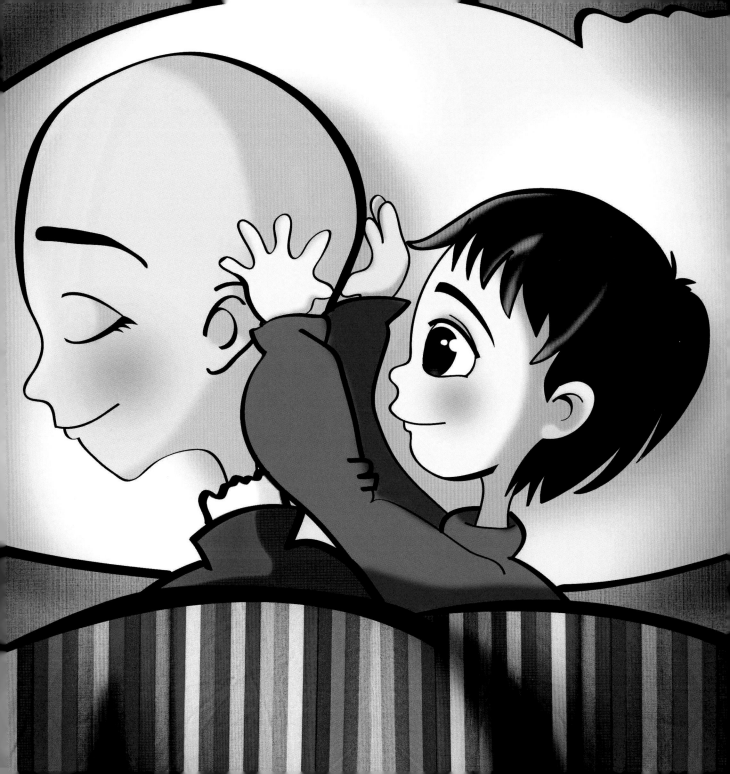

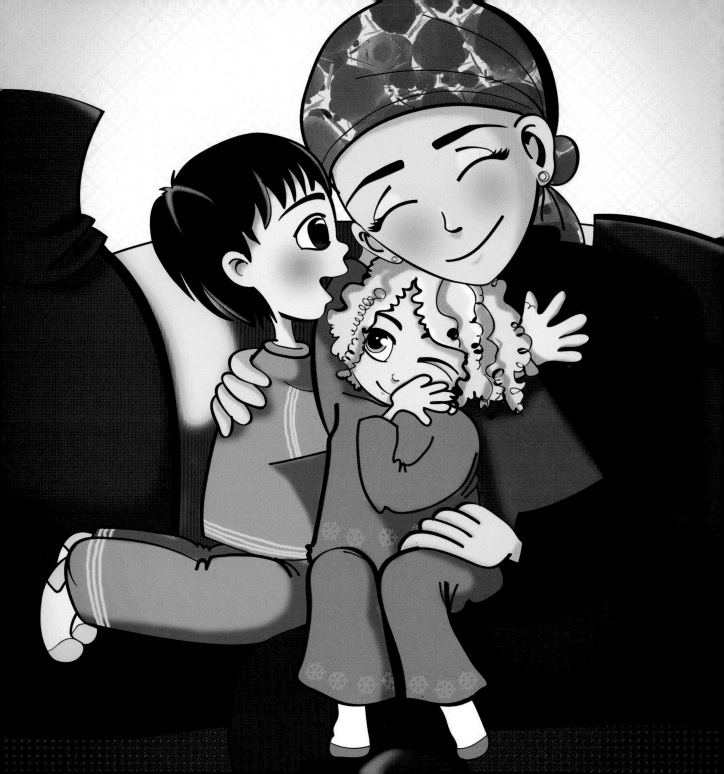

Mommy told me that her medicine, called chemo, was the reason her hair fell out. I realized that every time she got this chemo medicine she came back feeling tired and sleepy.

For a few days after my Mommy's chemos she felt really bad. On those days, we let her rest to help her get better and feel stronger.

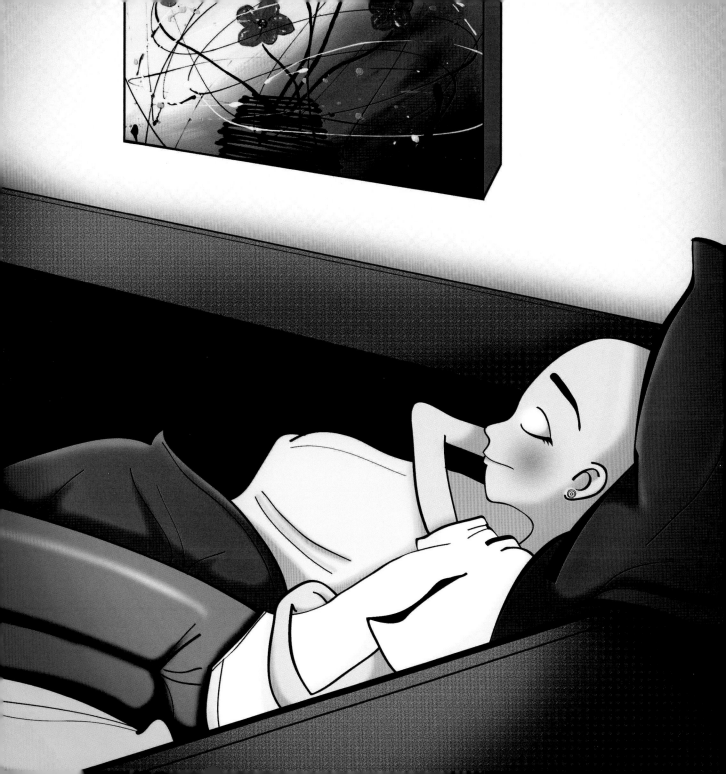

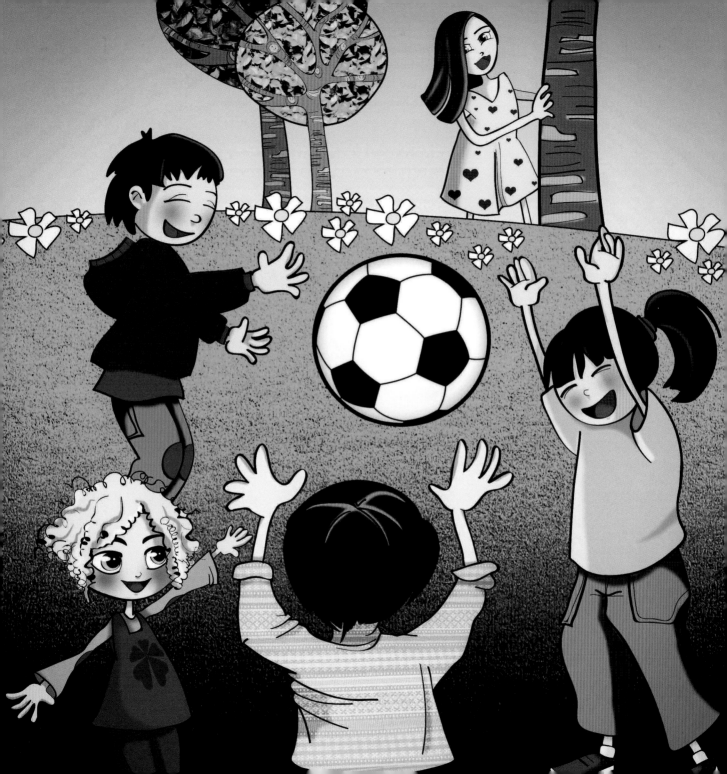

One of the things we liked to do on the days Mommy was sick was to visit friends and family. My sister and I sometimes went to our neighbors and had a great time. Other days we went to our friends' houses and enjoyed playing with them and their toys. We even went for sleepovers sometimes. I think we have the best neighbors and friends ever!

Another thing we liked was that we got to spend more time with Daddy. On the days Mommy was tired, he helped us get ready for school, made breakfast, and took us to the bus stop. That was usually Mommy's job. I missed my Mommy on those days but I was happy to be with Daddy too.

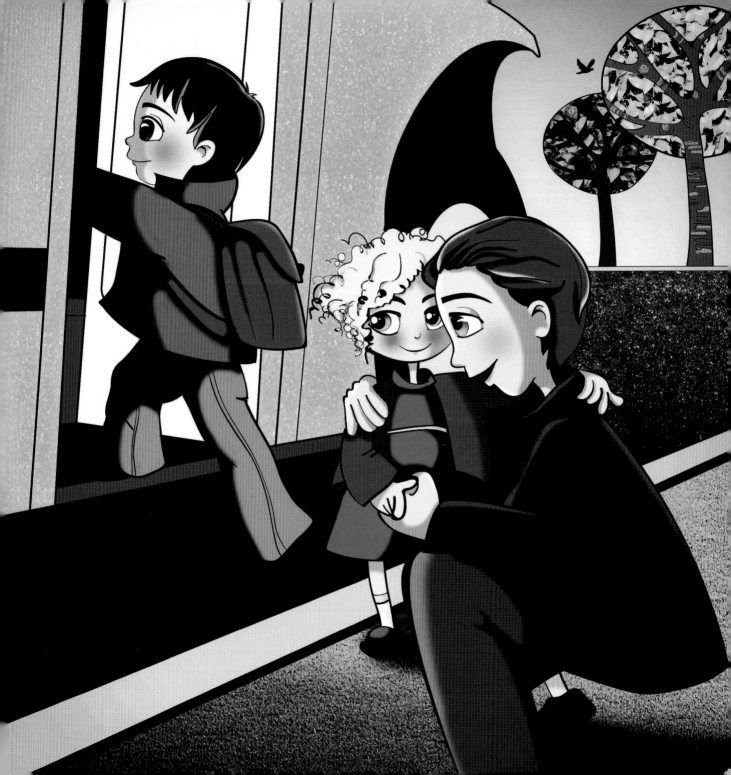

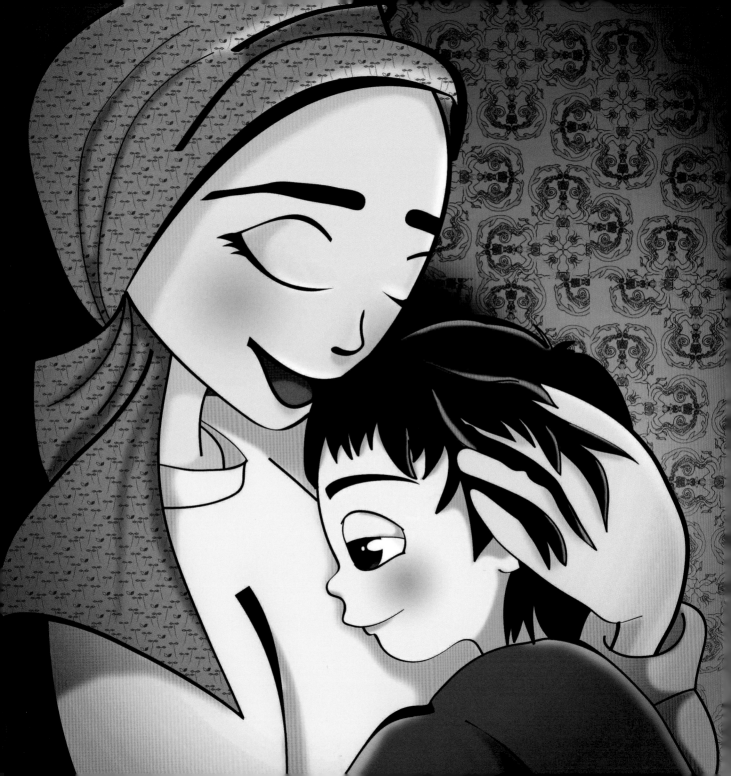

I was thinking about Mommy's cancer one evening before bedtime and I asked her: "What if your chemo doesn't work? Does that mean you're going to heaven like great grandma?" My mommy took me in her arms and said: "That is possible. Not all chemos work, but doctors have so many medicines and treatments I am pretty sure they will find the right ones for me."

Mommy also said I should never ever forget that God is watching over us. No matter what happens, He will take care of us. I have a good feeling we will be OK and I am so glad I asked this question.

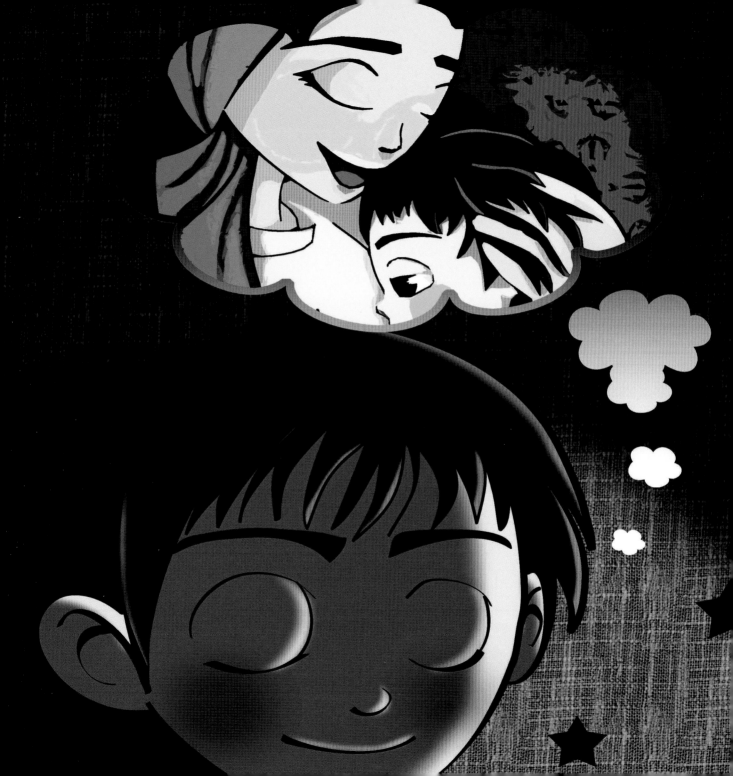

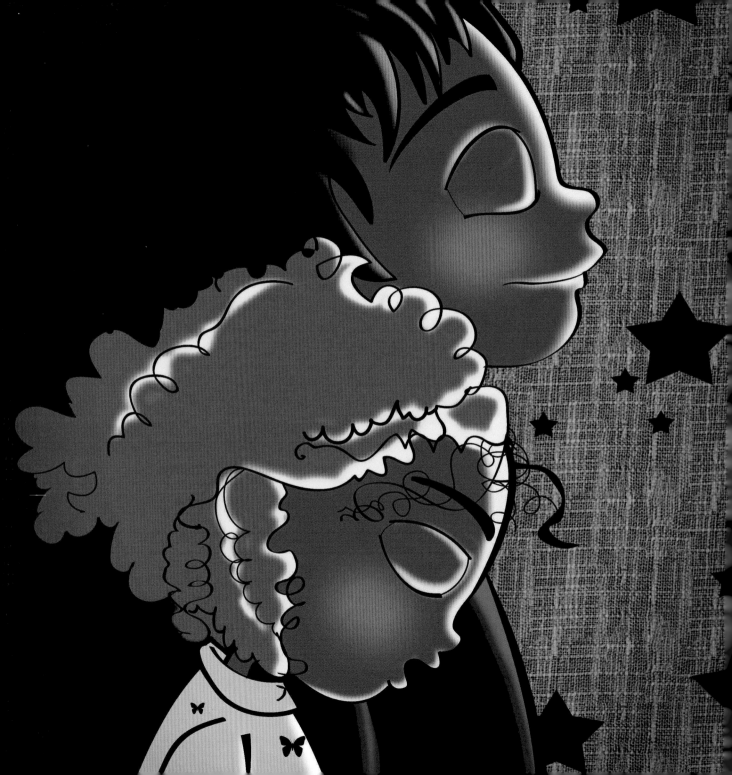

In the evening during prayer time, I always asked God that Mommy's chemo would go well and that her cancer would go away for good. My sister's prayer was to "let my Mommy's booboos go gone, Amen!"

I think God listens to us. I always feel better when I ask him to give me good dreams too.

Now I am older and we're further in the process. After her chemo treatments Mommy had surgery and radiation therapy, where the doctors took the rest of the cancer out. Mommy is feeling a whole lot better and her hair is growing back! Now she is able to do all the things we normally do. She is still going to the doctor and checking for cancer just in case, but I'm not as worried any more.

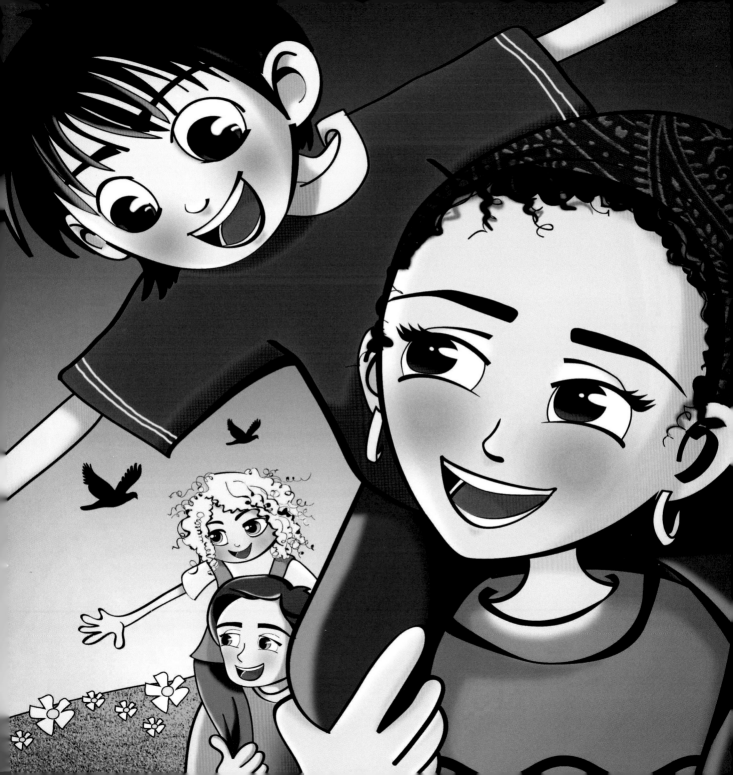

To my friends and family

My battle with cancer is not over. I am keeping my hopes up. Reaching out to my family and friends and getting this overwhelming wealth of support makes me feel blessed and loved, fortunate and happy. I want you to know that this disease will not defeat me, because God has blessed me with determination, hope, optimism and with YOU!

Jocelyne Smith
Mathuin's Mom